LIGHTER PRACTICE,

QUICKER RECOVERY.

A.D. TSWANYA MB.BS; Dip Derm.

MINERVA PRESS
MONTREUX   LONDON   WASHINGTON

LIGHTER PRACTICE, QUICKER RECOVERY
Copyright ©A.D. Tswanya 1995

All Rights Reserved

No part of this book may be reproduced in any form,
by photocopying or by any electronic or mechanical means,
including information storage or retrieval systems,
without permission in writing from both the copyright owner
and the publisher of this book.

ISBN 1 85863 363 X

First Published 1995 by
MINERVA PRESS
195 Knightsbridge
London SW7 1RE

2nd Impression 1998

Printed in Great Britain for Minerva Press

LIGHTER PRACTICE,

QUICKER RECOVERY.

*To Mom, Dad (of blessed memory),
and to the House officer, wherever he may be.*

About the Author

Abubakar Daniel Tswanya was born at Bida, Nigeria in January 1966. He studied Medicine at the Ahmadu Bello University Zaria; and pursued postgraduate study in Dermatology at the St Johns Institute of Dermatology, St Thomas's Hospital, London. He is currently a Medical Officer with the General Hospital Minna, Nigeria.

Acknowledgement

It has remained with me until this day, that Bello said, in unaccustomed words of 'prophecy' way back in 1990, 'We shall publish this in the UK someday!'

The amazement abides, that Mama studiously went through the complete manuscript on the eve of my departure to the UK, relishing even the risqué bits and saying, 'Abu, wannan ya yi kyau.'

Many were the friends and relatives who, reading the early bits and pieces of this book said, 'This is good. Beef it up and publish it!'

But for them, a long list, the printing of which will surely annoy my publishers, this book may never have seen the light of day!

Foreword

A sense of humour is an essential pre-requisite for most jobs and medicine is no exception. The long hours, the difficult decisions, the emotional atmosphere and the whims of the medical hierarchy all take their toll. Time for relaxation is infrequent and, therefore, precious. This collection of humour was devised over long weekends on call and late nights of duty. But in the same way that producing this book has helped the writer to unwind, reading it is also a great prescription for relaxation.

Roderick J. Hay FRCP, MRC Path
Professor of Cutaneous Medicine
St John's Institute of Dermatology
UMDS, Guys' and St Thomas's
London.

Dear Doctor,

If you see but a few patients and so can enjoy this book while at work, it must be a light practice.

If you keep patients waiting, to make time to peep into this book, ah-ah! – it's a sharp practice.

If you see patients and read this book at the same time, in other words reading and clerking together, it's malpractice.

If however you spend all day enjoying this book and not seeing patients, it's no practice.

If on the other hand, you spend all day and night with patients, and have no time for books such as this one, you must be the House officer!

This book is dedicated to the House officer wherever he may be.

A.D. TSWANYA MB.BS; Dip Derm.

Dear Patient

Laughter's the best Medicine. You may take an overdose.

A.D. TSWANYA MB.BS; Dip Derm.

Contents

Prologue	xii
Opening Remarks	13
Up the Walls	34
Money Talks	39
Different Strokes	42
Whys and Wherefores	50
Overheard	56
All in the Days Work	68
New Word Order	77
Closing Remarks	85
One Last Word... Er... Or Two	101
Epilogue	104
Appendix?	105

PROLOGUE

A jocose fellow walked into the Rimi Teaching Hospital one fine morning. He couldn't remember when last he'd needed a doctor. Even on this occasion, he only had an itchy skin lesion he couldn't just ignore.

'Next!' the doctor called out, and it was his turn to go in.

'Hi Doc, what's up?' he greeted.

Raising his head slowly, the look on his face serious, the doctor said in a rigid tone, 'Your time will come soon, if you don't just sit down. Now, tell me Mr Samson, how may I help you?'

Soon afterwards, and as a consequence of this episode, a graffito appeared on a wall in the hospital. It read:

WANTED.

HUMOUR IN THE HOSPITAL.

REWARD: LIGHTER PRACTICE,

QUICKER RECOVERY.

A chain reaction followed, like this:

Q. Why is everyone in this hospital telling jokes?
A. One good pun deserves another.

This book records it all.

OPENING REMARKS

Insomnia

Patient: I didn't sleep a wink last night.
Nurse: How could you have slept when you kept winking at me?

You're mistaken

Doctor: It appears you're scorbutic.
Patient: Not so, Doctor, I'm Punjabi.

Symptom

Patient: Doc, what's a symptom?
Doctor: A symptom is what the patient complains to the doctor about.
Patient: Well then, Doc, I have a symptom; you kept me waiting two hours.

Sit down

Midget: Good morning Doc.
Doctor: Good morning, Mr Simon, climb a seat!

Late

Patient: Good afternoon, Doc, sorry I'm late... say, what's up Doc?
Doctor: Your time. N-EE-X-TT!

The problem with specialisation

Patient: Doc, I've got an itch.
Surgeon: That's okay, we'd put a stitch.

Normal lifestyle

Doctor: Have you been leading a normal life?
Patient: Sure, Doc; eat, sleep, drink, smoke, women, late nights; see, all the normal things normal people do.

You have my word

Doctor: Promise you'll give up cigarettes?
Patient: I promise, Doc; as soon as I can afford cigars.

Easy

Patient: I've got a sore throat, I can't swallow.
Doctor: Well then, chew it.

Resignation

Psychiatrist: Who gave you the idea to come?
Kleptomaniac: I must have stolen it from my wife!

Resentment

Nurse: Do you have an appointment?
Patient: Yes, I paid for one.

Fish out of water

In the doctor's office:
Judge: This chair is most uncomfortable, Doctor.
Doctor: Nurse! His Lordship is used to the bench, get him one.

Side effect

Patient: Doc, I have a headache.
Doctor (pensive): Could it be the pill?
Patient: No Doc, I think it's the bill.

Mind your business

Nurse (passing by): Seen the doctor?
Patient (blind): No, only heard him.

Prurient

Chiropodist: What's your size?
Patient (preoccupied): Six and a half inches.
Chiropodist: I meant your feet, sir.

Thanks for sympathy

Nurse: Sorry sir, the doctor will not be available today. He's down with hepatitis.
Patient: That's okay, just show me who else to see.

Rash

Doctor: I'm afraid I cannot feel the lump.
Patient: I thought you wouldn't. It's on my head and not in my breast.

Better?

Doctor: How do you feel?
Patient: How else, Doc? With my hands!

Non-surgical

Patient: Doc, I feel like a can of worms.
Surgeon: Well, that's no reason to open you.

Eeeeeek!

Patient: Doc, I passed a worm in my stool this morning.
Doctor: Why are you so alarmed, did it say 'Hello'?

Rational man

Doctor: Do you drink?
Patient: Nope. Bad for the liver.
Doctor: Do you smoke?

Patient: Bad for the lungs.
Doctor: Do you womanise?
Patient: Bad for my wife!

That makes the two of us

Patient: Doc, I've got a pain in the neck.
Doctor: Mine just left, she's off to get the children from school.

Let's celebrate

Patient: Hi Doc, I've come to tell you I've finally given up booze.
Doctor: Congratulations, Mr Ivory. I suppose we can drink to that!

No love lost

Nurse A: The matron just slipped from the stairs and hit her head against the concrete.
Nurse B: That sounds serious! What happened to the concrete?

Tit for tat

Doctor: Why in the world did you do that?
Patient's Husband: Well, it's unfortunate Doc, it's just that she broke my heart and I broke her arm.

Sssssssshhhh!

Patient: And one more thing, Doc, the other doctor recommended I eat plenty of beans.
Doctor *(puckering his nose)*: That's all right, I got *wind* of it.

Fungus

Doctor: (Looking between child's toes) Your son has got athlete's foot.
Child's Mother: That's quite correct Doctor, he's on the school relay team.

Alcoholic?

Psychiatrist: Do you have a drinking problem?
Patient: Not at all, Doc, I've never had problems swallowing liquids.

Four too many

Outside the Labour ward:
Midwife: Congratulations, Mr Edwards, your wife just put to bed five lovely babies.
Husband *(startled)*: Five!... ehm... please tell her I'm off now, I'll be back when there's only one.

Fence

Diplomat: Can't you do better, Doctor? Your chair is most uncomfortable. I'm not used to anything like this.
Doctor: Sorry your Excellency; if I knew you were coming, I would have made you a fence to sit on.

Not alone

Patient: One more thing, Doc, my wife thinks I'm some kind of a meathead.
Doctor: Oh, she thinks so, too?

Last in line

Proctologist: Next!
Patient: Good afternoon, Doc, it appears I'm last on the poking order.

Risk?

Doctor: It's only a minor procedure, Mr Jacobs, but refusing Surgery puts you at great risk.
Aged Patient *(huskily)*: Risk? With all due respect son, I was stuntsman for forty years!

Middle of the road

Nurse 1: Hardly anyone speaks well of Dr Andrews, but what do you think?
Nurse 2: Let me put it this way, I see some method in his madness and some madness in his methods.

First things first

Patient: My teeth's aching.
Dentist: Very well then, to which do we attend first, teeth or grammar?

Two too many

Midwife *(radiant)*: Congratulations, Mr Fairweather; triplets!
Mr Fairweather: Good Gracious Lord! There goes Sally again, immodest as ever.

Not quite

Doctor *(looking at multiply bitten patient):* A neighbour's ferocious dog, I suppose?
Policeman: Not quite, Sir, his wife.

Not exactly

Doctor: The patient was hit by a truck?
Chaperone: Not quite Doc, beaten by a weightlifter.

Tall order

Nurse *(passing by):* Do you need a hand Doc?
Nephrologist: I'd rather a kidney, my dear. This patient needs an urgent transplant.

Trim

Dietician: We must cut down on everything, Susan.
Patient: Does that include the fee?

How come?

Doctor: You've got Crohn's disease.
Kleptomaniac: But how could that be, Doc? I never took anything from Crohn.

Confession

Patient: She's my twin sister.
Doctor *(rubbing his eyes)*: Thank God for small mercies, I almost started cursing the bartender.

Say that again

Doctor: It's so sad, the patient on bed six just kicked the bucket.
Nurse *(French)*: Ah! Cheer up Docteur, 'e would only 'ave ze sore foot, n'est-ce pas?

Aetiology

Lady: I've got an ache in the region of my heart.
Doctor: Who caused it?

Me too

Patient: Doc, I've got a nagging headache.
Doctor: I've got one too, she's at home.

In short

Patient: Is that to say my legs will never be equal in length again?
Surgeon: I'm afraid that's the long and short of it!

Case

Lawyer: Those terminology's are more than I can comprehend, could you give me the gist of it.
Doctor: Certainly barrister, I was only making a case for the amputation of your diseased limb.

Wrong number

Vigorously scratching his hand, a Gynaecologist consults a Dermatologist:
'My fingers itch, Jane.'
'Itch for what?' the hitherto distracted Dermatologist questioned amazedly.

What cheek

Nurse: Mr Williams, you've been on it for close to an hour, are you now through with the bed pan?
Patient: Oh, of course Nurse, you can now have it; and... er...*Bon Appetit*.

Any hope?

Psychiatrist: How's your memory faring now?
Patient: I cannot remember.

Better be sure

Doctor: Yes, Mr Smith, can I help you?
Patient: Well, if you're in doubt, I'd go somewhere else.

Can't be serious

Patient *(alcohol laden breath)*: Hi Doc; I've given up drinking.
Doctor *(puckering her nose)*: Now let's see... may I take a guess?
Patient: Sure Doc.
Doctor: Your tongue is in your cheek.

Can't say more

Psychiatrist: How exactly are you feeling now?
Patient: Peculiar.
Psychiatrist: Try. Can you improve on that.
Patient: If I could, I wouldn't have come.

Half an eye

Hypochondriac: Nurse! Nurse! It's all gone dark. I'm blind; I'm blind!
Nurse: That's a pity, Mr Willy. If you had half an eye you would've noticed the lights go off.

Mind your language

Nurse: Good morning, sir. Do you wish to see the doctor?
Blind man: No my dear, I only want his audience!

Indefatigable

Consultant: You hadn't a tie on yesterday because you had a sore throat; your buttons were undone because you were feverish; perhaps if I now asked why you haven't opened

your mouth all day to contribute to this tutorial, you'd tell me lockjaw?
Med. Student: Not unrelated sir, a mild trismus!

Consistent

One ward matron complaining to another:
Matron 1: Staff Veronica never does things the easy way.
Matron 2: I'm not altogether surprised; old habits die hard. Even at birth she was a breech.

Optimism

Nurse to patient with broken legs:
Nurse: How are you doing this morning?
Patient: Kicking, Nurse, thank you.

Mmmh... Mmmh...

Nurse 1: Dr Lucas must have very poor vision. I can tell by the thickness of his lenses.
Nurse 2: True; but *I* can tell from the look of his wife!

Doctor says

Patient: Nurse, how am I faring?
Nurse: Very well, Samson. Doctor says you're improving.
Patient: Nurse, may I have something to eat.
Nurse: Oh, of course. Doctor says you can now start taking orally.
Patient: Nurse, when can I see my mum?
Nurse: Soon. Doctor says you may now have visitors.
Patient: Nurse, you're so sweet. What does Doctor say your name is?

Spice

One patient to another:
'I never find that doctor's word palatable.'
'You would, if you took it with a pinch of salt.'

Had it

Patient (**For the umpteenth time**): Doctor, am I going to die?
Doctor: Unfortunately not, Mr Singh!

Obliging

Doctor: Why are you taking your clothes off?
Lady: But Doc, you asked to see my credentials!

Square one

Psychiatrist: How is your memory now?
Patient: Improved; and tremendously too, I must add.
Psychiatrist: Can you remember our discussion last week?
Patient (amazed): Oh! Were you the one I saw last week?

Gratis?

Doctor: I'm afraid, just as the other doctor said, the disease is advanced. At this stage there's little anybody can do.
Patient (depressed): I've heard that before.
Doctor: I suppose all that is left is to make the most of your remaining days, before the Good Lord calls.

Patient: I knew that before.
Doctor *(moved)*: I'm sorry.
Patient: You said that before.
Doctor: For me, no charge.
Patient: That I've never heard before!

Back to sender

Outside a doctor's office:
Husband: The Doctor says I have Piles.
Wife: Piles of what?
Husband: He didn't say; he saw it through the proctoscope!

Nothing to chance

Surgeon: The operation comes up tomorrow. Who would sign as next of kin?
Patient: Herbert.
Surgeon: Your husband?
Patient: No, my lawyer!

Stasis

Patient *(hoarse)*: Doc; I lost my voice.
Doctor: Beg your pardon, son; speak a little louder, I'm hard of hearing.

What it takes

Two kids, meeting in a hospital lobby:
James: My father is a psychiatrist. It sure takes a mind to be one.
Peter: My father is an abdominal surgeon. It sure takes guts to be one.

Waiting

Doctor (shaking a thermometer): Your temperature's pretty high.
Patient: Yes, Doctor; waiting makes my blood boil.

Far gone

Patient: Doctor, I don't seem to remember anything. I forget as soon as I know.
Psychiatrist: Calm down, Mr Longman. Tell me, for how long have you had this problem?
Patient: What problem?

Parkinson

Doctor: You have Parkinson's disease.
Lady: Yes Doc, and I think I have his baby too.

Not that you... !

Venereologist: Did you notice anything after you had sex with her?
Patient: Yes, Doc; my wallet got leaner.

Back to owner

Doctor: I'm afraid you have Hansen's disease.
Patient: That's okay, he can have it back.

Grrrrrrrrr!

Doctor: Good morning, what's wrong with you?
Patient: That's for you to say, Doc.
Doctor: Sorry then, what's your complaint?
Patient: I've been waiting to see you too long.
Doctor: No, no, I mean your reason for coming to hospital.
Patient: To see a doctor.
Doctor: Okay. Now that you've seen the doctor, what have you to say?
Patient: At last!

In a moment

Patient (reluctant): But, Doctor, would it hurt?
Gynaecologist (wielding an instrument): I don't know, but we'll soon find out.

What position?

Patient (mounting the couch): How do you want me, Doc?
Doctor: The sunny side up will do, Miss.

Insight

Patient: Doctor, I really don't know why I'm here.
Psychiatrist: Well, I suppose that's why you're here.

Holiday mood

Doctor (tugging child's eyelids): It appears your son's a little pale.
Mother: You think he needs a suntan?

Poison

Alcoholic: Is there anything wrong with my blood?
Doctor: I wouldn't say, but let's put it like this; if I were a vampire, I wouldn't drink it.

One last thing

Patient (reading out prescription): Antibiotics, vitamins, liberal fluids, anything else Doc?
Venereologist: Oh yes, my dear, prayers!

Helping hands

Wife: Darling, did you hear the doctor say I'd need absolute rest?
Husband: Yes, darling, but I didn't hear him say who would do the chores.

Beg your pardon

Wife: He's such a good doctor. He's so good with his hands.
Husband: Good at what?

Distrustful

Nurse: Come closer, let me take your pulse.
Patient: Where are you taking it to, Nurse?

Different strokes

Patient: Doc, my sleeping is excessive.
Doctor (looking worn out): I wish I could have just some of it.

Up

Patient: Hi Doc, what's up?
Doctor: Not much Peter, just the fee.

Contact tracing

Venereologist: Your partner would have to be treated too.
Lady: That's okay, Doc, but first I must consult my diary.

Strain

Doctor: It's a hernia. Do you carry heavy objects?
Patient: Yes, Doctor, my husband is close to a hundred kilograms.

How come?

Doctor (pointing to large sore on patient's phallus): You didn't mention that; where did it come from?
Patient: The Bristol Hotel, Doc.

Take it or take it

Patient: Doctor, I don't think I can stand the pain.
Doctor: Well then, let's try it sitting down.

It's an emergency

Nurse: Where are you off to, Doc?
Surgeon: To the Theatre.
Nurse: May I come along.
Surgeon: Sorry, no extra tickets.

Virus

Nurse: Do you carry your mini computer everywhere you go?
Kid: No, Nurse, we're both afflicted. I've got a cold, and it's caught a virus too.

Fine?

Doctor: How is it this morning?
Patient: *It's* fine I guess, but I'm not!

Manners please

Telephone Operator (harshly): Who are you and where are you calling from?
Psychiatrist (calling from the Psychiatric ward): I am Dr Abraham, and I'm calling from where you should rightfully be.

Touché

Patient: Seven hundred dollars for a minor operation? Are you kidding, Doc?
Doctor: Nope. And you ain't bidding either!

Extinct

Doctor with daughter in his office:
'Daddy, where does one get Chicken pox?'
'From a virus, and not a chicken darling.'
Five minutes later:
'Daddy, where does one get Small pox?'
'From the archives darling, from the archives.'

Venue

Doctor: That'll be all for now; next appointment, Thursday week 9 a.m.
Lady: Fine, Doc; your place or mine?

Heavyweights

Doctor: You have a pain over your sternum. Do you carry heavy weights?
Lady: No Doc *They* carry me!

Rehydration

Doctor: You are a little dehydrated.
Alcoholic: Not to worry, Doc, a bottle or two should sort that out.

Generous

Doctor (looking at chest radiograph): It appears you have a large heart.
Patient: That's interesting Doc, perhaps that's why we get on so well.

One way or another

Venereologist: Mr Valentine, the last time you were here you said it will never happen again. You promised to be circumspect about your choice of women.
Patient: That's true Doc, but you see, I was careful about choosing them; they weren't careful about choosing me!

Couch language

Doctor (*palpating patient's abdomen*): Does it hurt?
Patient: No.
Doctor: Here?
Patient: Nope.
Doctor: And here?
Patient: Not quite.
Doctor: Here?
Patient: O-U-C-H
Doctor: Now you're talking!

Always a reason

Doctor: It's not easy coming to terms with the fact that one would never walk again. I must remark, however, that you're taking it very well.
Paraplegic: Thanks for the encouragement, Doc The truth is, before my accident I went into a lot of debt, promising to pay back 'when I'm on my feet'. Now I don't have to worry about when that will be!

UP THE WALLS

Hospital Charges were recently reviewed upwards. The development wasn't quite welcome. Someone expressed his displeasure on the hospital entrance sign:

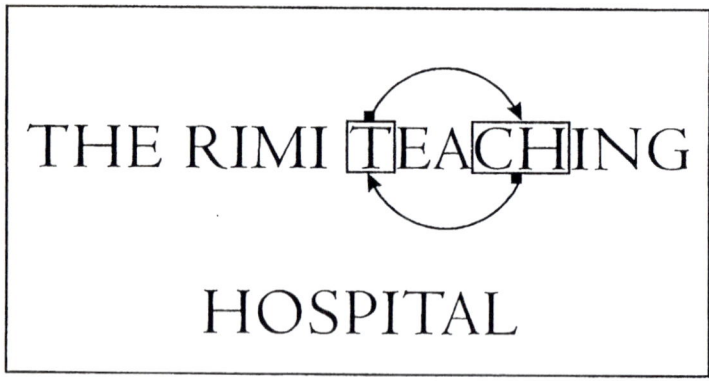

Labour ward graffito:

Eve, I hate you;
Adam, you shouldn't have listened.

Sign hanging on a Gynaecologist's office wall:

'Not mixing business with pleasure.'
Where could it be more pertinent?

Graffito on a GOPD wall:

Doctor, I'm ashamed of you.
                              Signed
                              Hippocrates.

On a wall in the hallway:

They say the Doctor's calling is humoneytarian.
I think so too.

Below it was another:

We are patients, not customers.

On a Gynaecologist's office wall:

I wouldn't know where life began.
It could have been in Egypt, the Middle East,
East Africa or wherever.
For all I care, it still begins in the pelvis.

On the theatre entrance:

Why do surgeons wear masks?
I don't know, I've never smelt their breath.

On a corridor wall close to the hospital Cashier's box:

Down and out
The illness the former,
the bill the latter.

On the GOPD exit:

Prayer and pill must go together.
You've only seen the Physician
and not the Prognostician.

On hospital toilet wall:

Traveller's Disease
How did Diarrhoea
beat Gonorrhoea to it?

On another toilet wall:

Disease Prevention is:
Good medicine,
Bad economics;
For the private practitioner.

Near a venereologist's office door:

Dear Doc

My father always told me not to take things from strangers.
I didn't listen, and that's how I got gonorrhoea.

Sticker on a Gynaecologist's door:

I love my job

Who wouldn't?
(Hand-written addition)

Revised Versions:

Prevention is better than cure
If you won't do it for your health
You'll do it for your money.

Health is wealth
You'll believe it when you see the hospital bill.

What a man can do, a woman can also do, but she would need a prosthesis.

To err is human. Doctor, it's your insurance.

A beggar has no choice.
The Doctor's worse off, he must treat friend and foe alike.

Practice maketh perfect.
Doctors practise all their lives; they never get perfect.

Out of sight, out of mind.
Sounds like a blind psychotic.

If you really think the law is an ass,
see a proctologist when you have problems with it.

All work and no play,
makes Jack a respectable gynaecologist.

Charity begins at home.
It never makes it to the hospitals these days.

Pride comes before a fall.
The doctor comes after the fall.

An apple a day keeps the doctor away?
Not when you owe him!

If at first you don't succeed, try, try and try again.
Sounds like a surgeon soon to lose his clientele.

True love is in the heart.
The myofibrils couple all the time.

MONEY TALK

From physicians to fee-sicians.
From wards to wads.
The more things change,
the more they aren't the same.

It's no more physician-patient relationship.
It's feesician-paytient relationship.

If money is your problem
see a doctor and he'd
take away your problem.

Doctors had made it known long ago,
It's your money or your life.

Doctors' fees don't help stomach ulcers and blood pressures.

What you pay the doctor these days
you'd've paid for the doctor those days.

There are two types of doctors,
The fee-type and the fee-type.
(Dr and $r. respectively)

I'm no longer sure what doctors are after nowadays,
saving life or life savings.

The doctor gave a clean bill of health – $1000.

Money talks, my doctor listens.
Doctors take my pulse but leave my purse.

What didn't the surgeon do?
    Cut corners.
What happened to the patient?
    He squared up.

The feeling's rife. Doctors' bills should be vetoed.

How to get more doctors into congress?
Raise the bill.

Who passes the bill?
    Congress.
Who pays the bill?
    Patients.

Labour Ward graffito:

Mom's in labour, Dad's paying the doctor.
No wonder new born babies cry.

Etched on the kidney transplant unit entrance:

God loves a cheerful giver.

Sign in an operating theatre (written by the Chief Surgeon):

To Err Is Prison

Near a paediatric ward:

Children like to play 'Doctor'.
Adolescents play Gynaecologist.

Title of an article on the hospital general notice board:

Manpower shortage in the Nursing services Department.

PS (hand-written)

Train more male nurses

In the Housemen's restroom:

Housemanship domesticates; taken too far, hospitalizes.

Bill on a surgeon's office wall:

Physicians make differentials.
Surgeons make the difference.

On a Physician's wall next door:

Of the noble professions were three,
Physician, Priest and Scribe.
The Surgeon was never listed.

DIFFERENT STROKES

On a busy surgeon's office door:

If you don't know why you're here, don't waste my time.

On a Psychiatrist's two doors away:

If you don't know why you're here, come in.

On the hospital main entrance:

Silver or Gold have we none, just sick people.

A snake, around a torch of flames. It reminds me of the Devil, how he first appeared and where he'd end up. How come it's this hospital's logo?

Ad. for a multivitamin capsule:

A CAPSULE A DAY
KEEPS DOCTOR AWAY

PS (Hand-written):
So Does My Doberman

Bill stuck onto a Hospital Friends Committee donation box:

I can't afford a dime.
At least I give a damn.

Sign on a dietician's office wall:

'Just a snack' and here you are.

On the X-ray Unit entrance:

Just a minute,
and we'll see through you.

Sign on a Plastic Surgeon's office door:

Designer looks? Inquire within.

Sign on the wall of a bifurcating corridor leading (Right) to the X-ray Unit and (left) to the Gynae ward:

>   Right ------------ > X-Ray
>   Left --------------- > X-Rated

On the Doctor's common room walls:

Physician heal thyself?
Nope, I'd seek a second opinion!

Spare the rod, spoil the child.
>PROVERBS

Spare the rod, stop Child Abuse.
>PAEDIATRICIAN

Spare the rod, and you may not make children.
>GYNAECOLOGIST.

Doctors are overworked.
Surely I've heard it before
'Physician kill thyself'

On a GOPD Clinic wall:

To stay healthy
I've given up
all that makes me happy
No thanks doctor.

Caption in the child Nutrition clinic, promoting Breastfeeding:

>BREAST IS BEST

P. S. (Hand-written)
>*I get the same feeling*

On a GOPD wall:

Surgeons are a scoffing lot. You should see what they call the Lord's procedure.

On a Gynae Clinic wall (by a male med. student):

Déjà-vu.
It was the feeling when I examined my very first gynae patient.

Notice on the maternity ward entrance:

CHILDREN BELOW THE AGE OF 10 ARE NOT ALLOWED INTO THE WARD.

PS (Hand-written)
    You'd be surprised what they already know.

PS (In a child's handwriting)
    I came, I saw, I couldn't believe it.

Scribbled close to a Gynaecologist's couch:

GUN SCARE
Be careful as you palpate, doctor,
She could be carrying a revulva.

On a Venereologist's office wall:

There's nothing private about those parts while you're in here.

Graffito close to the hospital pharmacy:

I hate tablets

P. S.   *Go on Moses, smash them.*

Popular Opinion.

For headaches, fever, aches and pains, take two tablets three times a day. If symptoms persist after three days, sue your Physician.

On a corridor wall:

I've never gained from this hospital.
I saw a Dentist, I lost a tooth.
I saw a surgeon, I lost an appendix.
I saw a physician, I lost a sum.

P. S.
> *But you lost your mind before you saw me.*
>
> Signed Psychiatrist.

If Doctors had business minds,
None would preach disease prevention.

On a Surgical ward:

My surgeon's generous.
Even with his scars.

On a Medical ward:

Mitral Incompetence?
The Bishop must hear this.

On the microbiology Lab:

Whoever named it 'Hookworm',
was never an angler.

On a wall in the speciality clinics:

I don't see my GP anymore.
I've cut out the middleman.

PS
> *That's okay, when you have a headache, go straight to the brain surgeon.*

Sign on a bald Dermatologist's Office:

THE LORD IS MY BARBER

On a GOPD wall:

The Doctor's job must be easy.
After all, the patient gives him all the clues.

On a wall in the operating theatre:

Inside Out;
only a surgeon knows you that well.

Sign on a busy out-patient clinic wall:

ALWAYS CONSULT A DOCTOR
YOU HAVE NOTHING TO LOSE

PS (Hand written)
> *But precious hours*

On a wall in a Psychiatric ward:

The world's gone crazy. I'm with it.

On a Dentist's office wall:

Supernumerary Teeth?
Make up your mind where you belong – Man or Crocodile?

Sign outside a busy Optician's Office:

Remain Patient. Don't make a spectacle of yourself.

On a hospital cashier's door:

After the fever, now the feever.

On a Laboratory wall:

Fungus A: I am being candid. Fungus B: I'm candida.

Outside a doctor's office:

Diminutive Dr Price must have a very high IQ. Pity he can't reach it!

On an operating theatre wall:

If, 'a-' means without, and
aesthetic means 'of the sense of beauty'
Anaesthetic = without a sense of beauty.
No wonder it puts everyone to sleep!

On a Psychiatrist's office door:

Come let's talk. One MD to another.

(NB. MD stands for (i) Doctor of medicine as well as (ii) Mentally Deficient.)

If you don't read graffiti, you may miss signs like this:

MIND THE GLASS

Concerned about the 'outbreak' of graffiti on its walls, the hospital authorities put up notices in large print on all corridors and wards:

POST NO BILL

Below one of such notices, someone inscribed:

My doctor still mails his.

WHYS AND WHEREFORES

Q. Why is a Dermatologist a friend to cherish?
A. He never gets under one's skin!

Q. What else goes up and never comes down?
A. Hospital bills!

Q. How can you tell a surgeon from a physician?
A. One stands longer than he sits, the other sits longer than he stands.

Q. Why is everyone running away?
A. Someone mentioned the doctor is 'dressed to kill' today.

Q. Housecalls, what do they achieve?
A. Home budget deficits.

Q. Where do you find long IQs (Eye Queues)?
A. Waiting to see the ophthalmologist.

Q. Where would you find a psychotic?
A. Round the bend.

Q. Why do doctors charge fees?
A. They haven't found a cure for it.

Q. What's to the surgeon as is to the singer?
A. Theatre.

Q. What is a Dermatologist hardly ever told?
A. 'Quickly Doc, it's an emergency'.

Q. Where was the first successful surgery performed?
A. Genesis 2:21

Q. What's the difference between a cripple and a Gynaecologist?
A. One walks on crutches, the other works in them.

Q. Where is the other Broca's Area (speech Centre)?
A. The United Nations.

Q. How do you know the surgeon hates his guts?
A. He yanked them out.

Q. Where's the Brain Surgeon?
A. At the headquarters.
Q. Where's the proctologist?
A. Hindquarters!

Q. How can you tell the Gynaecologist is not in a mood to work?
A. He wouldn't stir a finger!

Q. When does a woman attain men-no-pause?
A. When at 50, they still come after her.

Q. What's the difference between a diagnosis and a prognosis?
A. The doctor would rather the latter came after his bill has been settled.

Q. Where do they say doctors now worship?
A. At the shrine of Mammon.

Q. Why are you tremulous each time you're about to take that medicine?
A. It's on the bottle, SHAKE BEFORE USE.

Q. What comes between the 2nd and 3rd stages of labour?
A. P-U-S-H!

Q. Which is the most useful part of a stethoscope?
A. Between the two earpieces.

Q. What would a Psychiatrist call a patient who wouldn't respond to therapy?
A. A hard nut to crack.

Q. Why did Hitler never need a Cardiologist?
A. They say he was a heartless man.

Q. How did she get pregnant?
A. She skipped the morning-after pill.
Q. How did he get the scar on his face?
A. He skimped the morning-after bill.

Q. What happened to *free* medical Service?
A. The 'r' vanished.

Q. What happened to the baby who survived three months in an incubator?
A. He became the toast of the hospital.

Q. What happened to the man who thinks he's a dog?
A. The Psychiatrist unchained him.

Q. What's the difference between a Golfer and a Gynaecologist?
A. One's looking for a hole in one, the other knows exactly where to find it.

Q. How did the relatives recognise the patient who fell in the cinders?
A. The nurse gave a glowing description of him.

Q. How come she's so good in Osteology?
A. Everyone says she keeps a skeleton in her cupboard.

Q. What's the difference between a Psychotic and a Neurotic, Doc?
A. See I'd tell you; the psychotic refused to pay my bill, the neurotic paid twice.

Q. What did the Judge say to the Gynaecologist?
A. Do you swear to tell the truth, the hole truth, and nothing but the truth?

Q. Why is the Dentist like a bat?
A. He's always exploring cavities.

Q. When does Doc become Duck?
A. When he starts talking about his bill.

Q. Why do you address him as 'Dear Doctor'?
A. His services don't come cheap!

Q. What did the tapeworm say to the hookworm?
A. Caught any fish lately?

Q. When will you be thinking of taking a wart to a Psychiatrist?
A. When he's your impossible son.

Q. Why are frogs not welcome in hospital?
A. No one wishes patients to croak.

Q. What part of the brain would an Accountant want to know about?
A. The cerebellum. It keeps the balance.

Q. What can a short sighted patient see better than anyone else?
A. He can see why he needs glasses better than anyone else.

Q. Why would Gynaecologists make bad boxers?
A. They'd always go below the belt.

Q.	Why do patients not make acquaintances in the Gynaecologist's Surgery?
A.	They are always feet apart.
Q.	How's the heart unlike the abdomen?
A.	Soft is the heart when tender; rigid is the abdomen when so.
Q.	Why's the Ambassador's buttock sore?
A.	He's been sitting on the fence all day.
Q.	Why's the patient looking so flat?
A.	She's been under a doctor all day!
Q.	What's wrong with the carpenter?
A.	He has a mallet finger.
Q.	What did the obese acupuncturist complain of?
A.	Pins and needles.
Q.	What's with the jockey?
A.	He has a saddle nose.
Q.	What's happened to the Chef?
A.	He suffers the consumption.
Q.	What's wrong with the archer's son?
A.	He has bow legs.
Q.	How's the escapologist's condition?
A.	He's neither here nor there.
Q.	What about the violinist?
A.	He's fit as a fiddle.
Q.	Why is there such a high turnover in the skin's Malpighian layer?
A.	The one on top of it is a horny layer!

Q. Why does the medulla feel short changed?
A. Because the cerebellum keeps the balance.

Q. What's the eye's biggest disappointment?
A. Its pupil has not graduated all these years; and may never do!

Q. Why did the patient pass away?
A. To prove he was dead serious!

Q. What skin condition reminds many an employer of something she'd want to squeeze?
A. Fiddler's neck!

Q. Why may the liver ache towards the English Midlands?
A. It doesn't like the sound of 'Liverpool'.

Q. Why has Granny purchased ten cats?
A. Because the doctor called the sore on her face a 'rodent ulcer'.

Q. Why must dermatologists explain carefully to patients?
A. Not everyone thinks along the same lines when doctor says, 'You'd require a prick test for this, Sir.'

Q. What would you call it: the dermatologist offered sweets to the atopic infant who'd been wailing all morning?
A. Cry-o-therapy!

Q. Why does that psychiatrist irk the cardiologist next door?
A. He claims to be a mender, even of broken hearts!

OVERHEARD

'I wanted a prescription to empty my bowels, the doctor gave me one that emptied my pockets!'

'The doctor said that the IUCD failed. I disagree. I think my child was just determined, and he made it.'

Venereologist to Patient:
'You got involved with a carpenter's daughter?
Lucky, this time you have a sore on your thing; next time you could have a saw on it.'

'One always believed that the future of the world lies in the hands of men.
Now one gets the feeling it lies in the use of condoms.'

'The ward matron reserves beds 6 and 7 for the difficult cases – those that keep the doctors at sixes and sevens.'

'Medicine has advanced a great deal. Now, doctors can make the blind see, the lame walk, the deaf hear and the dumb speak. But still only a few are able to say to their patients, "Go, your bills are forgiven."'

'I've always said my wife was possessed. The doctor confirmed it, she has worms.'

Said a grieving widow:
'Herbert was such a Zealot. The doctor only said he'd require a lot of rest, and he passed away.'

'The doctor told me that in smoking or giving it up, the choice is clearly one between life and death. I told him I'd settle for life after death.'

'If with all these symptoms, the doctor still thinks I'm a *hypo*chondriac, I'd hate to see what 'chondriacs' look like.'

'Dr Bright has a superb diagnostic acumen.
He can tell when you've not settled his fees, from a mile.'

'In the past, doctors were hardly ever free. They were either on the wards, or headed for the wards. Now, take away the *r* from *free* and *wards* and you know where they're headed.'

Child pointing at a passing Psychiatrist's jacket: 'Mom, is that why he's called a shrink?'

Patient to Psychiatrist:
'I told my wife that after 20 years, I am in love with her anew; she said I could tell that to the marines.
The next time I said it, she said I could tell it to the Pope. When I said it the third day, she said it's time to tell it to a doctor, and I'm complying, Doc'

Embonpoint

Doctor to obese patient:
'Good morning madam, take a seat... er... er... or two.'

'Having paid so much for consultation, the doctor comes to ask: "And how are you feeling this morning? Of course, run down."'

Physician heal thyself.

Doctor to patient:
'Oh Hell! I know I'm a very patient doctor, but this is the eighth time you've made me swear in thirty minutes.'

Said an ailing patient:
'The hospital charges are killing. I never complain out loud, but each time the cardiologist listens to my heart, he picks the murmur.'

'There goes my doctor, you can see he's well looked after.'

Said a Physician: -
'She came in pain, excruciating pain. Quite tender with guarding. Acute abdomen, no doubt. An itchy surgeon, true to type, went in. Finding no pathology, took out her appendix. He called it exploratory Laparatomy, I'd call it burglary. If he had taken his time, he would have diagnosed mittleschmertz.'

'I have read pieces like:
'he is the architect of his fortunes'
'he engineered this success story'
'our company midwifed other successful ones'
'God is my only advocate'.
I have also read pieces like this:
'the study was a fiasco, the figures were doctored.'
Someone does not like doctors.'

'Dr Hope's approach must be working.
In just a week, I have lost a hundred pounds. One tenth in flesh, the rest in cash.'

'I went to the dentist for a denture.
It appears he gave it to me without the -ure.'

Said embittered lady to doctor about her ex-husband: 'Encephalitis? John? I thought it could only happen if one had a brain in the first place.'

Market strategy

Said a class teacher of his doctor:
'I saw my doctor the morning I had an itch on my foot. He gave me a cream and suggested I take the day off until it was over.
I saw my doctor the morning I felt terrible from a "hangover". He suggested I went straight back home, and nowhere near school.
I saw my doctor the morning I came down with a bad flu. He gave me Vitamins, something for the headache and suggested I went straight back to class.
I couldn't understand why, but he sure had a pleasant look on his face when I brought seven of my pupils to his consultation next day.'

'She walked in looking sick, and walked out looking chic. He is either a good doctor or a sweet talker.'

Doctor to Reverend (not regular with his drugs):
'In Hospital we say "non-compliance"; in Church you say "backsliding". The wages are the same, Father.'

'I heard the surgeon say I'd be all right. I suppose he's not wrong after all.
Having amputated both left limbs, I guess I'm all right.'

Alibi

Alcoholic to Doctor:
'It works very well for my colds and cough, more so I don't like syrups.'

Two to tango

'I could have sworn it wasn't there this morning,' said man to psychiatrist, of his wife who thinks she's lost her head.

'Dr Andrews saved my life. But that was more than he could do for my life savings.'

Said an Accountant:
'I complained to my doctor about a persistent headache. He prescribed some medicines, advised I slacken a bit on the job and recommended physical exercise.
Smart guy, he knows I'd be back with a backache.'

Said a Geriatrician:
'Such is the case with my patients, the memory gets shorter, the stories get taller.'

Brevity of life

'The doctor said I'd need this medicine for the rest of my life, but he prescribed enough to last only a week!'

Patient to wife:
It's so good to see you darling. You're the only one around here who takes me for what I am. To the nurses, I'm "bed number 17". The medical students say I'm "an interesting case" for discussion. The consultant thinks I'm "good teaching material" and the professor thinks I'm "publishable stuff" for the big journals.

'He's been acting different since his chest Operation. He despises friends, disowned his daughter and ended his thirty year marriage to Evelyn. The surgeon must have tampered with the bottom of his heart!'

Lawyer to Doctor:
'Sure, I've been examined by the doctor next door. I've only come here for cross examination.'

A Gynaecologist boasted:
'Of course I'm well looked after. A full wife at home, mid-wives at work.'

Side comment as an anaesthetist addressed a gathering:
'Y-a-w-n... ! Did Dr Jones bring his gasses along?'

News from the hospital grapevine has it that a nurse jilted that Dermatologist for a Cardiologist. Said she:
'I've had enough of the surface, I wish to go deeper.'

Knock 'em off

Said of a Dentist:
'He is an old hand. First as a schoolboy, then an amateur boxer and now a dentist.'

Venereologist to Juvenile:
'Be more circumspect young man. I wouldn't want to see you clapped in here any more.'

Exasperated surgeon to unyielding motor mechanic: 'I'm afraid, gentleman, to save your life, that limb must go. Pity we don't stock spare parts here.'

Gynaecologist welcoming new set of medical students to the department:
'While you're here, you may hear all evil, see all evil, touch all evil, but take no advantage.'

Psychotic to Psychiatrist:
'Honestly, Doc, I'm beginning to think our thoughts correspond all the time.'

Foley catheter.

A nurse to other, on the circumstance of a patient's injury: 'I still cannot understand why he took such a risk just to impress those girls. Now he's injured and has ended up with a folly catheter.'

Said a Physician whose office had been burgled:
'Our surgeons are talking plenty about "keyhole surgery". I would assume it has nothing to do with picking locks!'

Patient to Gynaecologist:
'When I said,"I still feel the prick from time to time", I was referring to the pain and not what you are thinking, doctor!'

Foreign patient introducing interpreter to doctor: 'She, Rosalyn. She, my hearing aid.'

Dentist to unwilling patient who shut tight his mouth at the approach of the drill:
'I take no pleasure in doing this, my dear. It's most unlikely I'd strike oil in there.'

'Dr Jeff has appeared in court five times on malpractice charges. On all occasions, he's worn the same pair of jacket and trousers. It appears that's his malpractice suit.'

'Doctor says no more booze, no more smoke, no more women, no more butter, no more cheese and no more eggs. He says, that way one could get a few extra years but it sounds to me like polite euthanasia!'

Venereologist to Patient:
'Your girlfriend was here yesterday; she had a vaginal discharge. In just *one* word, tell me Peter, how do you plead, guilty or not guilty?'

Said a lawyer:
'I never appreciated the value of Locus Standi until I sat before a doctor with my wife, listened to him ask her very personal questions, and found myself not in a position to say 'objection Doctor.''

'A child does not do well at school; beats up colleagues, and is rude to teachers. As his doctor, I'd want some assurance he's not just a chip off the old block!'

'Why do some doctors now insist on "pay before service"? Well it's like this: you rid a patient's knees of arthritis, he refuses to pay because now he can stand up for his rights.'

'My doctor was quick to point out that women were the source of my problems. She advised I gave them all up and kept to my wife. I did, including her.'

'In my practice, I try to cure my patients. I have no business trying to please them. The years have taught me to make it so. Now you have an overweight patient complaining, "Doctor I look awful, I feel terrible. I get embarrassed everywhere I go."
Soon she'd be saying, " ...and where the hell does he (the doctor) think I'd get the money for new slim-fit clothes?"'

Said of a Psychiatrist:
'If truly doctors learn from their patient, Dr Wood has learnt a lot.'

'As the gynaecologist examined me, the thought kept coming like a scratched record: "This is private property; trespassers should be prosecuted... This is private property... "'

Child to mother:
'Mom, "he has a finger in every pie"? Is he a gynaecologist?'

Patient to venereologist:
'Doctor, I hate to be referred to as gentleman! If I were, I wouldn't be here.'

Midwife to pot-bellied man:
'In case you need me, call my number.'

Patients to Doctor:
'Doctor, are you sure I'm getting better?'
'Doctor, don't you think I'd require a second opinion?'
'Doctor, you promised I'd be out of bed in a week. It's eight days now and I still can't budge.'
Nurse (under her breath):
'All they're asking is value for money.'

'My husband's knees got swollen; the doctor called it "Bursitis". I asked him to "say in English" what that meant. He called it the "Housemaid's knee". A timely clarification stalled a divorce suit.'

'Doctor says it's because I worry too much. Doctor never says it's because I'm paying too much.'

Patient to Psychiatrist:
'I'm not going to answer any more of your questions. I'm sure Doc; you'd find me a hard nut to crack!'

'My doctor reminds me of my wife.
"Don't do this, don't do that; no more this, no more that; cut this, cut that out."'

Who, me?

Nurse to frightened patient, waiting to see the doctor:
'Relax Mr Stevenson, there's nothing to worry about. Dr Lawson wouldn't hurt a fly!'

'I have one good reason to be happy – that now I'm well. My doctor has three – that I'm well, it's good riddance and he's richer.'

Man to doctor:
'You asked if my wife has put to bed; well she did more than that, she put to three beds.'

Blockhead

'The brain Surgery lasted ten hours, it appears the surgeon left no stone unturned.'

Nurse to Patient:
'You may eat all the beans in the world, Mr Frank. I'm anosmic.'

Said a Surgeon's wife:
'It was a wonderful Saturday evening. My husband and I enjoyed 'theatre'. I watched ballet, he watched a thoracotomy.'

'Nobody thinks I'd ever have anything of my own. Even the doctor says I have a pigeon chest.'

Just doing his job.

'My doctor drinks, smokes and drives like a maniac. Yet he never stops telling me what to do or not do, to live long.'

'I am 18. The doctor says I have measles. That's no diagnosis, it's an anachronism.'

'My doctor's full of sugary talk. He forgets, I'm diabetic!'

Said an accountant:
'The doctor keeps assuring me that mine is not a terminal disease, but I still cannot understand why he insists on his bills settled up front.'

'Each time I see Dr Matthew, I'm not sure what to call myself – James or Guinea pig!'

A Child's definition of Doctor:

'A doctor is a person who treats sick people and takes money from them.'

Said a Psychotic:
'Of course I'm a very important personality. I get more death threats than the president of this country!'

Psychiatrist (foreigner) to patient:
'You say it rain "cats and dogs" that night?'
'... I see... ' (scribbles it down) '... Hallucinations!'

Husband to wife:
'An apple a day keeps the doctor away? Darling, send him one everyday until we're able to settle his bill.'

Said a Houseofficer of his Consultant:
'Dr Cook is tough. Each time he comments on one's performance, he seems to take the wind out of one's sails. When for once he commended me this morning, it sure took the wind out of one's self.'

Cold War

Physician to Patient:
'I agree you should also consult a surgeon. You'll never live to regret it.'

'The way that Psychiatrist keeps harping on about my son's 'split personality', I think I know where he's headed – a fee for each person.'

Priorities

'I was very ill but the doctor didn't quite say of what. All he told me was that I urgently needed an organ transplant. While he worried about finding a compatible donor, I worried about size.
The mention of "Dialysis machine" put me in the proper perspective.'

Indulging doctor to patient:
'I must warn you, my dear, alcohol is bad for your breath.'

Doctor to Patient:
'Once more, Mr Ivsky Krzyzewski, what's the problem, bowels or vowels?'

Tell it to the broads

Venereologist to teenager:
'You got it from a "toilet"? Is that what you call them these days?'

Doctor to child:
'You were bitten by an Adder? Gee, how's your Math then?'

Finito!

'The doctor called it Grave's disease. Why did he then bother to write a prescription?'

ALL IN THE DAY'S WORK

Squint

Both distracted by an immodestly dressed Nurse, a doctor and a visitor to the hospital bumped together on a corridor.
'Next time, Doctor, you look where you're going,' the visitor said, wiping his shirt.
Looking up and noticing the man had a squint, the doctor replied. 'And next time, sir, *you* go where you're looking.'

Fee

A private practitioner, wanting to remind an ex-patient to settle his fee, at the same time not wanting to seem importunate, wrote:

> *Dear Feelix*
> *Congratulations on your quick and complete recovery. I hope you enjoyed your stay in our hospital.*
>
> *Cheers.*
> *It's Feellip*
> *Your Feesycian.*

Physician heal thyself

Persuaded by incessant taunts from her pupils about her nose, a young school teacher decided to go in for a rhinoplasty.
On her first visit to the plastic surgeon's, she met a man with a similarly bulbous nose in the hallway. Rather indiscreetly she asked, 'Good morning, Sir, something tells me we're here on the same mission; could you show me to Dr Hussein, the plastic surgeon?' To her chagrin the man answered, *'I am Dr* Hussein!'

Bet

A midwife walked out of the labour ward, to an expectant father who had been pacing up and down the waiting room, biting his finger nails and muttering things to himself, in the last hour.

'Congratulations, Mr Allwell, your son arrived twenty minutes ago. Mother and child are fine,' she announced.
'I won. I won!' he exclaimed jumping and throwing his fisted hands into the air, 'She owes me a hundred dollars!'

Consistent

In the two days since her admission, the patient on Bed 8 had complained about everything on the ward-nurses' behaviour, doctor's lateness, uncomfortable beddings, prying inmates, cold food, on and on.
On her third day, just as the doctor's rounds were about to commence, she said, 'Good morning Doc; you're looking good today.'
'Thank you; and thank God for once you're not complaining,' the doctor was about to say when she added, 'But your necktie is rather loud.'

Not letting go easily

A young couple were bringing a domestic 'who rules' game to hospital as they argued over features of their new-born baby:
'The nose's mine; so is the mouth; well I'd concede the ears; and she's got my dimple too. That's three to one in my favour,' said the wife.
'No, no. You're concluding too fast. We can only tell as she grows,' the husband contested.
'No... No... No... blab... blab... blab!'
'Certainly not – please be reasonable.' They went on and on pointlessly, until they were interrupted by a loud fart, and then a generous spray of meconium all over the crib.
'Okay, I give up,' the husband then said, 'it's four to one in your favour; she has your character!'

Plus ça change...

Robert Bush left medical school at 23. Then, Bob gave way to Doc among friends. On the wards and hospital corridors, 'Good morning, Doc' 'Hello, Doc' 'See you in the morning, Doc' evoked in him some satisfaction.
As a resident, 'Good morning, Doctor', 'Good day Doctor', 'Hello Doctor' were no longer a thrill. As a consultant, many years later, the tone of salutation had changed – 'Good morning, Doctor Bush,' 'Good day, Sir,' etc, and he didn't have to reply all the time. A nod or wave in acknowledgement sufficed.
Now at 75, and as old-time Professor, he still waddles in and out of hospital. Age telling on his auditory apparatus, the same old salutations begin to sound like 'Good morning, duck,' 'Ha-llooo, duck', 'see ya in the morning, duck.' Little wonder he now insists, 'Just say Bob!'

What dose?

An outpatient doctor was notorious for his 'speed' in attending to patients – before you gave your complaint he's handed a prescription. He got the shock of his life the day he said to a patient who had brought her baby on follow-up, rashly as usual, 'Take a seat' and she asked having not quite understood, 'How many spoonfuls a day?'

Be my guest

As the Psychiatrist handed some sedatives to a patient's wife, he explained, 'Your husband should take one of these just before he turns in at night. If still he disturbs your sleep, be my guest.'
'Thank you doctor,' the lady said delightedly, 'but what's your home address?'

Sanity First

Lamenting the attitude of doctors towards patients, in the hospital, the Physician-in-Chief completed his talk saying ' ...and I pray that someday, we find ourselves in our patient's shoes.'
The Psychiatrist in attendance demurred most audibly!

Teething Problem

'Next!' and an old man in his eighties walked into the dentist's room to everyone's curiosity.
'Good morning, Pa. Sit down, open your mouth,' the young dentist said as was routine. 'But you haven't any teeth in there,' he further observed. 'I know son,' said the old man, 'I wan 'em back!'

Stitch

Usman and Francis, medical students on their surgery rotation, had dates for the evening. It turned out to be a very busy day in the operating theatre, and Dr Bullock, the team consultant, insisted they stayed around.
Close to teatime, Usman feigned a sudden abdominal cramp; that way he got excused and kept his date.
Francis wasn't so lucky. 'Bullock ruined my date,' he lamented much later.
'What a pity,' Usman sympathised. 'A stitch in time saved mine.'

Round the bend

A lady, visiting the hospital for the first time, met an attendant on the corridor and said;
'Good morning gentleman. It's taking me so long to locate Dr Dubbs, could you help?'
'Dr Dubbs... Dr Dubbs... you mean the psychiatrist?'
'Yes please.'
'That's no problem,' the attendant said pointing down the curving corridor. 'If you'd gone round the bend you'd've met him.'

Infraction

A middle-age policeman was rushed to hospital from work one morning. Having been resuscitated, his wife was led in to see him much later. Delighted to see her and eager to assure her his condition was 'nothing to worry about' he said, 'The doctor said it's only a mild Myocardial infraction.'
'Now, now, Solomon,' she cautioned, 'this has nothing to do with the Law. The word is in-farc-tion.'

Working too hard

Dr Hook, a gynaecologist, wouldn't believe his wife that he was working too hard until she complained that he'd been assuming 'a funny posture' in his sleep lately. Her description suited the lithotomy position!

Golden Rule

A young lady who was herself a Caesar at birth, just had her first child through a Caesarian section.
In a moment of pain post-operatively, she confided in a nurse about her son, 'I'll name him Confucius!'

Timing

In a week of his labour ward posting, Dr Silas had observed that more deliveries were taken at night than during the day. 'Have you ever wondered, Matron, why more babies choose to come at night?' he asked. 'Oh that's not hard to see,' the matron explained, 'most of them are made at night.'

For Mr, Please

Dr Arnold sent his bill to the employers stating inter alia, that Mr Smith, their staff had undergone surgery for a 'Right vaginal Hydrocoele'.
A week later the bill was returned, with the word 'vaginal' underlined in red ink; and an accompanying note read:

> *Dear Dr Arnold,*
> *We would be delighted if you would send us the correct bill for Mr* Smith.
> *Thank you*
> *I. J. Brown*　　　　　　　　　　*Managing Director.*

My Boss's Problem

A young resident in Psychiatry was running a clinic and got talking plenty with a new patient. At some point in their discussion the megalomanic patient remarked, probably in reference to a naevus on the doctor's face, 'Gee, Doctor, something about you reminds me of my boss.'
'I see. That's an interesting coincidence. Something about you too reminds me of my boss,' the doctor said, and lowering his tone added, 'the difference is that you've come for help, he still hasn't.'

Down Tools

'We're all going on strike,' the doctors agreed as their meeting drew to a close.
'We're dropping our knives,' emphasised a voice from the surgeons' corner.
'We're hanging up our stethoscopes,' a Physician chipped in.
An elderly gynaecologist, gesturing with his index and middle fingers, was heard to say, 'If that's the case, we'd keep our fingers crossed.'

Overdoing it

Mr Brown had never felt so babied, at 50. The nurse gave him a bib and cajoled him to eat. After the meal, she patted him on the head. 'That's a good boy.' She'd ask things like 'Do you feel like a warm bath?' 'You will remember to brush your teeth before you turn in, won't you?' and when he was asleep she came around to pull the sheets over him.
Early the next morning she was at hand to ask, 'Is there anything I can do for you, Mr Brown?'
'Oh yes,' he replied in a tone of sarcasm, 'maybe you'd want to change my napkins, I think they're wet!'

Tit

A young foreign dentist had problems making the 'th' sound. For instance, for 'Filth' he would say 'filt', 'Tenth' – 'Tent', and 'Teeth' – 'Teet'.
Although proud that he'd picked up the English language 'in record time', he was soon to realise how much work he still had to do on phonetics, when each time he tried to say 'show me your teeth,' many a lady would grab her breasts in alarm.

Where exactly?

Dr Matthew almost always came late for the weekly hospital interdepartmental meetings, as Tuesdays were his theatre days. If from a Laparatomy, he would excuse himself thus; 'Sorry gentlemen, I got stuck in the abdomen!' If from a chest operation, he'd say: 'Sorry gentlemen, I got stuck in the thorax.'
This Tuesday, Dr Harris, a gynaecologist, came late having just finished a colporraphy. His apology went thus, taking after Matthew's 'Sorry gentlemen, I got stuck in the... er... er... er... er theatre!'

Wages of thin

A Reverend gentleman made regular visits to the cancer ward to pray for the patients. On almost every visit he'd shed tears as he prayed. One day he confided in a faithful nurse who always consoled him as he wept. 'Nurse, do you know why I cannot hold back the tears each time I see these brothers and sisters thinning away?' he said wiping his tears. 'I'll tell you. They remind me of my congregation, it's thinning away by the week!'

Surgeon

An elderly lady went to a police station to report a break in.
'Can you describe the man who robbed you?' the duty sergeant asked.
'Yes, yes sergeant,' she replied eagerly. 'He was big, wore a mask and held a knife in his hand.'
Visibly disappointed, the policeman said, 'Is that all? For all I know, that could have been any surgeon.'

Whassat?

Mrs Shehu took Michael, her very reluctant son, to a dentist. As they sat waiting for their turn, an anguished yell 'O-u-c-h! O-u-chh!' came from the dentist chair. 'What was that?' Michael asked, visibly more frightened. 'It was the dentist,' replied his mother smartly, 'the patient must have bitten his hand!'

NEW WORD ORDER

Diarrhoea:
A bout in public spells 'Dire rear'.

A Grave Prognosis:
Speaks for itself.

Good for nothing:
A Surgeon lost both thumbs.

Mitral Incompetence:
The Bishop's bungle.

Mitral Insufficiency:
The Bishop needs more hats.

Hen-Pecked:
'Congratulations, Mr Parker, your wife just put to bed a set of quintuplets; all female.'

Patriotism:
'I'm afraid, Mr Kohl, it appears your son has German measles!'

Verbosity:
'The doctor says I have "Strep-to-co-ccal Pharyn-go ton-si-illitis" and all I have is a sore throat.'

Squint:
When one eye does not seem to know what the other is doing.

Skin Grafting:
Robbing Peter to save Paul.

Morbid Anatomist:
One who flunks all anatomy tests.

Dentist:
One whose designation should scare car owners.

'There goes Carol, she's a dentist.'
'I can see that, her car bears testimony!'

Psychiatrist:
One who, like everyone else, cannot say precisely where 'the mind' is located but is the one to find it when you've lost it.

Houseman:
Usually a nosocomial being.

Houseofficer:
The first line of defence.

Traumatologist:
Pick a bone, break a bone and you'd find out who he is.

Gynaecologist:
One who works where others play.

Surgeon:
One who often mutilates to mitigate.

'*Dr* Bello, you're a surgeon remember, not an interior decorator!'

Prosthesis:
What you need when yours ain't working.

Stretcher:
A piece of hospital equipment, guilty of false pretences. Over the years, it has made no one taller.

Kidney dish:
So-shaped, so-called, but may never get to carry kidneys.

Proctologist:
The man in-charge at hindquarters.

Stethoscope:
The Doctor's companion, the Pressman's counterpart. It reports every noise but only a little louder.

Morgue:
A transitory resting place for extinguished ladies and gentlemen.

Idiopathic:
A reminder that there's still work to be done.

Bill:
Now an iatrogenic problem.

Palpitation:
A concomitant of hospital tabs nowadays.

Hypertrophy:
An affliction of the Ego soon after medical school.

Atrophy:
An affliction of the young doctor's ego, who works all night, and feels his pockets in the morning.

Long Sightedness:
Not appreciating things close to one:
e.g. 'Dr Thomas didn't marry a doctor, he didn't marry a nurse, he married a lawyer!'

Litigation:
A useful tool in preventive medicine. It keeps down iatrogenic diseases.

Malpractice suit:
A euphemism lawyers use nowadays for 'let's share the spoils, Doc'.

AIDS Scare:
Projecting the condom as a 'saviour of the world'.

Hospital recovery:
Hardly ever complete. Just when you think you're there, the patient gets home sick, drug sick, nurse sick or hospital sick. One never gets well in hospital!

Medical Practice:
Everyone has heard how the surgeon gave the patient an ugly scar, but no one wants to hear how the surgeon caught hepatitis.

Nursing:
10.03:	'Nurse! Can I have the bed pan please?'
10.10:	'Nurse! May I have these bedsheets changed please?'
10.21:	'Nurse! May I have some water to drink?'
10.23:	'Sorry this is a bit too cold; could you make it warmer?'
10.30:	'Nurse! It is a bit warm in here. May I have the air conditioner on?'
10.40:	'Nurse! It's getting rather cold, could you lower the speed?'
10.45:	'Nurse! It's still too cool. Just turn it off, open the windows and switch on the fan.'
10.55:	'Nurse! It's about time for my medication.'
11.05:	'Nurse! May I have a hot cup of tea!'
11.07:	'Nurse! I forgot to say 'noire'; may I have another, please.'
11.10:	'On second thoughts I'll settle for coffee. Forget the tea!'

It takes a 'nurse' to be oneself at 11.11 a.m.

Anticlimax:
Surgeon: Phew! Done at last.
Nurse: Doctor, I've just realised we're one swab short.

Clerking:
Rote for the beginner.
Detail for the intern.
Summary for the Consultant.
Tiring for the patient.

Clerking (continued):
Med. Student: Do you often have a headache?
Patient: No, but I have one now.

Libido:
Keeps the world growing.

Lockjaw:
Afflicts the medical student who hasn't the answers to the consultant's questions.

Intersex:
A shot at 'self sufficiency'.

Transsexual:
God says, 'Thou art John.'
John says, 'Joanne I am.'

Morning Sickness:
The feeling one gets when one sees the workpile on the office table.

Condom Failure:
Some owe their existence to it.

Dominance:
A Y-linked trait.

Emancipation:
An X-linked advocacy.

Aids-Related-Complex:
The feeling that sets in when the news breaks out that he has AIDS.

'High' Fever:
What dope has afflicted on society.

Penile Envy:
Not purely a matter of 'yours is bigger than mine'.

Specialisation:
Q: Are you a doctor?
A: No. I'm a Cardiologist.

Alarmist:
'When I have a headache, I call my GP My wife calls the MP'

Antithesis:
'Granddad got so obsessed with growing taller, he shrank; and had to see a shrink.'

'Profound' Observation:
Surgeon: 'Oops! I must have punctured the aorta.'

Hypochondriac:
One whose symptoms span the specialities.

Health:
Most taken for granted. That explains all the fuss about doctors' fees.

Chivalry:
A Sign 'Ladies First' on a Gynaecologist's Office door.

Understanding Wife:
One who wouldn't object to her gynaecologist husband 'bringing work home from the office' while she's away.

Obstetric Analgesia:
Adding 'not necessarily' to Genesis 3:16.

Menarche:
Discovering *men*, she goes *anarchy*.

Menopause:
Men tire and they pause.

Amputation:
What the unscrupulous hopes would happen to the long arm of the law.

Chest pain:
What is suffered when the treasury runs dry.

Munchausen's Syndrome (Private practitioner's view):
The more the merrier, as long as bills are settled.

Medical Jurisprudence:
The Science that tells us how to get the doctor to jail, and hands him the keys.

ICU (I see you):
A place where the services must not blink.

Physician heal thyself:
Patient: 'Doctor, my son stammers.'
Doctor: 'I sss-suggest yyouu ss-see the ssspe-eech thhh-erapist nn-ext door.'

Tall Order:
'My wife's started complaining about my short stature. Do something, Doc!'

Cot Death:
Many a paediatrician would wish to command: 'Kid as you were!'

Proxy:
'Doctor, I don't get enough sleep at night; I'm badly in need of a sedative for my husband.'

Autodiagnosis:
'Doc, I have a pricking pain in the stomach. Give me something for pinworms.'

Casualty:
Judging by the number of patients coming in from Road Traffic Accidents, it should now be spelt 'Carsualty'.

Cost of Living:
What you paid the doctor who saved your life.

Hypnosis:
Sounds like what a patient said to a nurse he suspected was trying to seduce him
(HIP? No; Sis.)

No work done:
'I told the surgeon about my dandruff.'

Open Secret:
In a Psychiatric Ward:
'Nurse! Tell the doctor standing next to you his fly is undone!'

Wise stake:
'I promise, Doc; but if I don't settle your bills in a week, you may have my appendix.'

Physician's Might:
'Good morning, madam. Take your clothes off. Good. On the couch. Good. Legs apart. Good. That'll be all madam; your fee is a hundred dollars!'

CLOSING REMARKS

Haggling

Wife: How would it look if I argued a bit with the plastic surgeon to beat down his fee?
Husband: I don't know how it would look, but I can imagine how you will look after the surgery.

Doctored

Husband: Gee! You're already looking different.
Wife (Emerging from a doctor's office): Of course; I've just been doctored.

Rainy day

Psychiatrist: Why are you standing on one leg?
Patient: I'm saving the other for a rainy day!

Counterpart

Child (Going through a Surgeon's theatre photographs): My dad does these things too.
Surgeon: Oh I see, he's a surgeon too?
Child: No, he's a butcher.

Cut me not

Surgeon: What would you like to be when you grow up?
Child: One whole piece!

No love lost

Wife: That patient needs a heart transplant, and you think I'd make a good donor? What about me? How do I end up?
Husband: Just the way I want you darling; just the way I want you.

Suicidal

Son: Mom, Doctor says smoking is dangerous. How come he smokes?
Mother: I don't know, maybe has a suicidal tendency, that's all.

Ouch!

Son: Mom, what did the doctor say?
Mother: Not much; he made me do all the talking.
Son: What did you say?
Mother: Ouch! Ouch! Ouch! That's about all.

Angina

Husband (gripping his chest): Darling, it's the pain again. Doctor says it's Angina.
Wife (blasé): That's interesting, I always thought she was Florence!

Left handed compliment

Wife: Darling, am I the only sugar in your tea?
Husband (Diabetic): Sure you are Victoria, sure you are.

Guilt

Doctor: Did you take any medicine before you came?
Kleptomaniac: No, Doctor, was any reported missing?

Out of the bag

Child: What's that?
Ward Matron: It's a rectal thermometer, son.
Child: What does it do in the mouth?
Matron: It's not meant for the mouth, son.
Child: But that nurse put it in my mouth this morning.

Resentment

Doctor: Would you foot the bill?
Patient: Sure, Doc, you put it on the floor and see.

Resentment

Doctor: Did you foot the bill?
Patient: No, Doc, I kicked the cashier.

Pleased to meet you

Patient: Good morning, Doctor. I'm all aches 'n pains.
Doctor: And I am, Dr Stevens. What's your problem?

ENT

One patient to another:
'That's an Ear, Nose, Throat, doctor.'
'Gee, and what happened to his eyes?'

Sick

Doctor: Hello, my turbaned friend, are you Sikh?
Man: Not quite Doc, my daughter is; I'm well.

Your turn

Patient: Doctor, there's a sore on my foot.
Doctor: Let's take a look.
Patient: You do, Doc, I've been looking all day.

Dermatologist

'Hello there, are you a skin doctor?'
'No madam, I'm a skint one!'

No you can't

At 2pm:
Patient: Nurse may I eat?
Nurse: Of course, that's why you have a stomach.

At 3.15pm:
Patient: Nurse! Can I pee?
Nurse: Of course, that's why there's a toilet.

At 5.02pm:
Patient: Nurse! May I take a walk?
Nurse: Of course, that's why you've got legs.

At 9.05pm:
Patient: Nurse! May I now sleep?
Nurse: Of course, that's why you've got a bed.

At midnight:
Patient (winking): Nurse! May I ask something?
Nurse: Of course, that's why you've got a mou-u-th. I beg your pardon?

No dice

Dentist (looking into patient's mouth): One... two... Where's the third hole as you claim?
Patient: It's in my pocket. I lost my wallet on my way here.

Evident

Patient: Doctor, I am a little off colour today.
Doctor: I can see that, Miss Brown, the mascara's gone and the rouge's a shade lighter.

If you say so

Doctor: Now don't tell me you've not been taking your medicine.
Patient: I won't, Doc, you'd find out.

Bowels Movement

Nurse: Good morning, Mr O'Brian. Have you moved your bowels?
Patient: No, Nurse, they're still in my abdominal cavity.

You too

Nurse: You doctors are all alike.
Doctor: And you nurses are all I like.

Second opinion

Doctor: Have you seen the consultant?
Patient: Yes, Doctor.
Doctor: What did he give you?
Patient: He gave a second opinion.

Intact

Wife: You're different. What happened to your sense of humour?
Husband (just discharged from hospital): The doctor cured it!

Denial

Doctor: It looks like your son has scabies.
Lady (feeling slighted): Beg your pardon, Doctor, is that some kind of a joke?
Doctor: No madam, it's a skin disease.

Undercover

One nurse to another:
'Why is the policeman on Bed 6 wrapped under the bedsheet?'
'I can't say; maybe he's an undercover agent!'

Bar

Doctor: How long have you been drinking?
Lawyer: Ever since I was called to the bar, Doc.

Slimmer

Dietician: Are you Miss Davies?
Patient: I was. Now I'm half Miss Davies.

Manhole

Patient: Doctor, I'm hurt. I fell in a manhole.
Doctor: O – O! How did that happen, didn't he have his trousers on?

Crown

Husband: Darling, I'm off to the dentist to fit a crown.
Wife: I wish you luck, your majesty!

Prognostic factor

Teenager: Doctor, would I live to be seventy?
Doctor: Yes, you have a chance, if you'd just leave my daughter alone.

Not so fast

Patient: Doc, I think I'm cured.
Nurse: Wait till you've settled your bills. If you still feel well, then you're cured.

Plastic

Two kids meeting in the hospital lobby:
Tom: My dad's a Plastic Surgeon.
Peter: Oh I see, mine's a real one!

Dye

Patient: Doc What do you have for grey hair?
Dermatologist: Deep respect, sir!

Grrrrrrr!

Doctor: For how long have you had this pain?
Patient: Since I turned 21.
Doctor: When did you turn 21?
Patient: At the time the pain started!

To be sure

Matron (checking): Did the nurse on duty take your pulse tonight?
Patient (feeling his wrist): No, matron, it's still there.

Not that one

Doctor: Where's your pain?
Lady: He's waiting in the lobby.

Psychosomatic

Patient: Doctor, there's been no improvement. This pain in my thumb is getting out of hand.
Doctor: Sure it's out of the hand; it's in the mind.

Precaution

Patient: Doctor, what's my prognosis?
Doctor: First settle my bill, and then I'll tell you.

Delusion

Psychiatrist: Why are you making that noise?
Patient: To scare away my enemies.
Psychiatrist: But there are no enemies around here.
Patient: You see, it's working.

Halitosis

Dentist: I recommend this mouthwash to you. I use it too.
Patient: If so, no thanks. I'd try another one, Doc.

Clothes off

Psychiatrist: Why are you taking your clothes off?
Patient: So sorry. Should I be taking someone else's off?

All your life

Doctor: Had this skin disease all your life?
Patient: How do I know Doc; I'm not dead yet.

Source

Doctor (puckering his nose): Hmmmm! I wonder where this smell is suddenly coming from.
Patient: Search me!

Teeth not trousers!

Dentist: You'd require braces.
Patient: I don't think so. My trousers fit.

The show

Man: How are you so sure my wife's already in labour?
Obstetrician: Because I've sighted the show.
Man (now fisting his hands): Show? How many viewers were there?

Decided?

Psychiatrist: Is your mind made up?
Patient: No Doc, it's plain, no make-up!

Fowl

Dentist: Your breath smells foul.
Patient: Yes, that's what I ate this morning. A whole one.

Never sure

Psychiatrist: You say you never are sure about anything?
Patient: I think so, Doc!

Booze

Doctor: Do you drink?
Patient: Sure Doc, when I'm thirsty!

Dyspnoea

Doctor: Do you sometimes have difficulty breathing?
Patient: Yes Doc When there's a bad smell in the ambience.

Dyspepsia?

Doctor: Does your pain rise when you're hungry?
Patient: No Doc; my temper does!

Smoke?

Doctor: Do you smoke?
Patient: What brand?

Cough?

Doctor: Do you cough?
Patient: I don't. It comes on its own!

Deaf?

Doctor: Are you deaf?
Patient: You haven't told me.

Leave?

Kleptomaniac: May I leave your office?
Psychiatrist: I'd be obliged. Were you thinking of taking it away?

Aged

Doctor: How old are you, sir?
Octogenarian: Very!

Steps

Doctor: You've suffered this illness for about a year. What steps did you take before coming here?
Patient: The ones at the end of the corridor!

Drip

One patient to another:
'She can't move out of bed, the drip wouldn't allow her.'
'Which one, the nurse or the IV line?'

Terms

Surgeon: Now let's get this straight; I'd be paid in full if the operation is successful. What do I get if it's anything short?
Lawyer: Twelve months, at least.

Diet

Nurse: Did you follow the doctor's diet?
Patient: Yes I did. He has a terrible eating habit.

Any more

Doctor: You promised not to drink any more.
Patient: Sure Doc! I've kept to two bottles a day!

Knife

'I once lived on prescriptions.'
'When was that?'
'Before I became a surgeon!'

To the point

Psychiatrist: That'll be enough. Now, can you go straight to the point?
Patient: What point? I'm not going anywhere until I've finished talking; and you just listen to me Doctor!

Nuts

Patient: Doctor, I keep thinking I'm going nuts.
Doctor: Stop thinking; believe it.

Pain

Doctor: Are you in pain?
Patient (groaning): No, Doc; the pain's in me.

Eight pound

Midwife: Congratulations, Mr Isaac, your wife just had an eight pound bouncing baby boy.
Mr Isaac: Oh thank you Nurse, but I have no intention of selling him!

No beating

Psychiatrist: Has your husband been acting strange lately?
Woman: Yes Doc; he hasn't laid a finger on me in three weeks.

Worm

Patient: Doc, there's a worm in my leg.
Doctor: I see. Guineaworm perhaps?
Patient: No, Doc; Woodworm!

Silver spoon

'I tried to impress my doctor, by saying my son was one born with a silver spoon in his mouth.'
'Well then, was he?'
'Not quite. Rather he said I was lucky, the spoon could have caused lacerations!'

Dogs

Doctor: I'll tell you, anyone who drinks the way you do will always surely go to the dogs.
Patient: (Hic!) True Doc You're the third one I'm going to.

Heaven

Patient A: My Doctor thinks the world of himself.
Patient B: Mine's worse. He never stops telling me heaven helps only he who helps himself.

Non-committal

Patient (looking into the mirror): Huh. Doc! Is this my head?
Psychiatrist: Well, I wouldn't know, but it's the one you came here with.

Under?

James: Where's your wife?
John: She's under the doctor.
James: Doing what?

Rhythm

Patient: I was once a weak man.
Doctor: And now you're how-many-times-a-week man?

Watchman

Patient: Doctor, I've been watching my weight.
Doctor: I can see you're a good watchman. None's lost.

Animal lover

Nurse A: Dr James loves animals.
Nurse B: No wonder; he works like a horse, drinks like a fish and walks with feline grace.

Capsule

Psychiatrist: Take this capsule everyday.
Patient: How? I'm not an astronaut.

Language

Orthopaedic Surgeon: But what's the bone of contention?
Gynaecologist: I really cannot put a finger on it.

ONE LAST WORD...
ER... ER... ER...
OR TWO

You tell the Paediatrician your son's 'fingers are all thumbs'; and he's thinking of a rare congenital anomaly.

Mention to the Psychiatrist how it 'rained cats and dogs' the day you left home; and he'd think you were hallucinating.

Talk about 'having a finger in every pie'; and the Gynaecologist will think you are referring to him.

If you thought you had left nothing out by 'starting from scratch' the Dermatologist will tell you, you still left out the itch.

If word goes around that you are 'cutting your teeth' on some new endeavour, the Dentist will already be expecting you.

If it is said that someone 'has made an ass of himself' the Proctologist may feel obliged to go check him over; or 'he has made a spectacle of himself' and the Optician begins to stir.

In criticising a doctor's judgement you would prefer 'prejudiced' to 'jaundiced' as the latter could have many a Physician peering into eyes.

Even at the height of exasperation, never say to a surgeon 'cut it out'; he may just reach for his knife.

In case you wish to discuss PR with any Doctor, first be sure his mind does not go to the rectum.

'There's no cure for this disease' does not write off bills.

'There's nothing to worry about' does not include the doctor's fee.

'Will it hurt?' A silly thing to ask the doctor; ten to one he hasn't tried it on himself.

'Doctor, am I getting better?' You can be sure he'd tell you what you want to hear.

Being in them or tending to them, long queues are one dislike patients and doctors have in common.

After Housemanship, only two letters matter – G and P. One either goes GP or PG

Doctors are the worst patients and patients are the best doctors.

Nurse patients well or nurse conscience so.

In the Doctor-Patient relationship 'The Fee' is central. If the doctor is not talking about it, the patient is complaining about it.

Consider this:

'Oh that's my doctor.'

'Meet Dr Matthews, our family Physician.'

'She has an appointment with her Gynaecologist.'

'His Surgeon thinks it's not time to take out the appendix.'

'Have you been seeing *a* Psychiatrist?'

'*The* Psychiatrist thinks he needs further therapy.'

Hardly anyone would address a Psychiatrist with possessives!

EPILOGUE

Jocose Mr Samson came back to see his doctor after a week, on a follow-up appointment. The itching had subsided and the lesion was clearing.

'Next!' the doctor called, and he went in.
'Hi Doc, what's up?' he greeted.
Slowly raising his head, the doctor answered, this time with a smile on his face, 'The spirits, Samson, the spirits!'

This Book Does Not Have
An Appendix.
It Saw A Surgeon Before
The Publishers!